One Mother's Journey

Creating My Family through In Vitro Fertilization

BY JENNIFER PRUDENTI
WITH JANELLE JOHNSON

WESTBOW PRESS
A DIVISION OF THOMAS NELSON & ZONDERVAN

WestBow Press books may be ordered through booksellers or by contacting:

WestBow Press
A Division of Thomas Nelson & Zondervan
1663 Liberty Drive
Bloomington, IN 47403
www.westbowpress.com
1 (866) 928-1240

ISBN: 978-1-4908-8397-7 (sc)
ISBN: 978-1-4908-8395-3 (hc)
ISBN: 978-1-4908-8396-0 (e)

Library of Congress Control Number: 2015909424

Print information available on the last page.

WestBow Press rev. date: 07/14/2015

This book is dedicated to my Angels on earth, Michael and Sophia; Marty, the one man who always stands by me, and to the millions of women that are out there striving for Motherhood.

CONTENTS

PART TWO: BUNS IN THE OVEN

PART THREE: THE FANTASTIC FOUR

Foreword

I remember when Jennifer wound up in the hospital on bed rest. I remember talking to her on my way home from the office. She was hysterical. She was scared. And all she wanted from me was reassurance that she- and her babies- would make it home. Healthy. I really just listened and talked her through all of the chaos that was going on. But in my heart I knew she and the twins would all make it home healthy. I just knew it. Just like I knew she'd get pregnant. Just like I know this story- Jenn's story- needs to be shared. More stories like this need to be shared. Countless women are struggling to conceive yet so many of them only share their stories behind closed doors. Jen is bringing her story to you to share and to bring hope. In my clinic I have witnessed too many woman facing fertility challenges and too many woman holding back their stories. I would love to see more women share what they went through to conceive and how they got their healthy babies home.

Prologue

My journey to give birth to my beautiful twins Michael and Sophia was one characterized by multiple setbacks, steely determination, mind numbing disappointments and inimitable joy, so in other words - an eventful one. Obviously, I didn't conform to the typical course of baby making and I feel that it is imperative that I provide you with some background about the events and choices that inevitably led me to the point of having to embark on this IVF journey.

Every woman has a unique story to tell about their voyage to motherhood. My hope is that by relaying some of these intimate details that people generally do not share, that you the reader, can take note of pitfalls you can avoid that may eliminate your need for IVF in your future or at the very least prepare you for demands that this journey will elicit from you if you do decide to take this route. I feel that for me to speak honestly and completely about my journey, it is important that I start from the very beginning of my process. So here is some insight into the multitude of decisions and consequent results that launched my rite of passage into motherhood.

I grew up in the Bronx, Throggs Neck to be exact, as the only child in a single parent household. I could never remember being miserable during my childhood, but I could also always recall feeling that there was a void in my life that I could never fill, and it came down to not having a dad in my life. I can only imagine the heartache my mother felt when every Christmas at the top of my list to Santa I always had daddy written in all caps. No other toys held as much importance to me as getting a daddy. This is not to say that I did not adore my mother and had a very happy childhood with her, and I know that some kids are just fine being an only child with just one parent, but I always missed having that father figure in my life, even though my Grandpa was always around, it's different..

So it would come as no surprise that I developed some major "daddy issues" like so many other girls out there. This in turn led me to seek out approval and love from just about every boy that I dated. In my mind every boy was "the one" and every relationship was going to inevitably lead to marriage. At age 14, I could clearly envision being married by 22 and having a child by 24, along with the house and white picket fence - you know, the whole nine yards. Wow, what a reality check I was in store for...

I had sex at a young but fairly average age, which I think was average for my time, my neighborhood and most of the girls in the neighborhood. Don't get me wrong, some of my closest friends didn't have sex until much older and some of them even married those guys (and are still married!). That's not my story...

For me, sex was a way to "get the boy" and I guess you could say I was somewhat promiscuous (this is the part where people that *really* know me may chuckle and say *somewhat...*). In addition, when I was young, protection wasn't something that I really thought too much about, and therefore was not something I employed on a consistent basis. Well, at 17, I got pregnant and it wasn't by a boy that I was dating but rather a boy that I had literally thrown myself at. For me at that age, keeping it was not even an option, nor was I going to attend school while pregnant and then give the baby up for adoption. So, I made the momentous decision to have an abortion, and even worse, to keep this decision a secret from my mom – an unfortunate lapse in judgment that I would later come to regret.

I went to a Planned Parenthood clinic in a Bronx hospital which didn't require parental permission and I distinctly remember it being one of the worse days of my life. First of all, "Papa Don't Preach" by Madonna must have actually played in the waiting area about 25 times during the six hours I was there. You could look around the room and see the twisted torture you felt reflected on each girl's face, it was just terrible.

The procedure itself was relatively quick and then I was on my way, with a follow-up appointment scheduled for the next two weeks. Of course real life soon intervened in the form of a graduation present from my mom - a trip to California and Hawaii, which meant that I never made my follow-up visit within the two week time frame. I was able to make my follow-up visit four weeks later. It seemed to be a routine visit with no issues being raised by the doctor who saw me. So I went on my merry way thinking that this ordeal was fully behind me. Unfortunately, I was not quite so lucky. Not even two months later I began experiencing excruciating cramps and incredibly heavy bleeding. My mom was of course very concerned and immediately took me to the emergency room. Of course I had no choice by that point but to finally come clean and let her know what had occurred, since I had to relay this information to the admitting nurse. My mom was devastated, not by the fact that I had become pregnant or had elected to have an abortion, but because I hadn't shared with her the ordeal and I had gone through it by myself.

From this experience I learned that I had contracted Chlamydia (curable but with ensuing damage) from the boy who had impregnated me. This in turn had messed up my fallopian tubes quite badly. Not only were they severely infected, but they were blocked as well. At this point, my mother took me to see her doctor, whom I will call Dr. Joe, the man who would later deliver my beautiful twins Michael & Sophia. Dr. Joe informed me that at this juncture with the damage that had been done to my tubes, with one being completely closed off and the other severely blocked, I had approximately a 1% percent chance of ever becoming pregnant in the future. While this certainly sounded daunting, becoming pregnant was not something that I was concerned about at that time so I could not fathom the full implications of this diagnosis.

Fast forward a few years into the future and I am in a serious relationship. My boyfriend and I had been dating for a few years in a monogamous relationship and we came to a decision to stop using condoms since we were committed to each other and there was no chance of me getting pregnant anyway. Of course you know full well where I am going with this don't you? One constant in my life was the fact that my menstrual cycle is completely predictable. In fact it would not be a stretch to say that my periods always came like clockwork, right down to the hour! So when I was late I immediately knew that something was up, I took a pregnancy test and then the improbable news was revealed that I was in fact pregnant.

I tried to grasp how this could even be possible after having been told how unlikely this scenario could be and I reached out to Dr. Joe for some explanations. After submitting to another test, this time using a blood sample, my pregnancy was confirmed. I was then sent for a sonogram which in turn determined that my pregnancy was stuck in my fallopian tube and I had an ectopic pregnancy, which needed to be terminated immediately.

In a normal pregnancy, a fertilized egg travels through a fallopian tube to the uterus where it then attaches and starts to grow. In an ectopic pregnancy, the embryo implants outside the uterine cavity, primarily in the fallopian tubes. Such a pregnancy is a potential medical emergency due to the risk of internal hemorrhage that can be life-threatening.

An ectopic pregnancy is usually caused by damaged fallopian tubes. Contributing factors usually range from smoking, to a pelvic inflammatory disease arising from an infection such as Chlamydia or gonorrhea, endometriosis which causes scarring in or around the fallopian tubes and being exposed to the chemical DES before birth.

Although a urine test can show if you are pregnant, for an ectopic pregnancy your doctor will likely do a pelvic exam, a blood test that checks the level of the pregnancy hormone (hCG), a test which is repeated two days later, then finally an ultrasound can be used. Common treatments are the administration of medicines, in most cases methotrexate through one or more shots, or through surgery called a laparoscopy if the pregnancy has gone beyond the first few weeks.

Dr. Joe reassured me that the termination of the pregnancy would be a simple out-patient procedure - a laparoscopy, where there was no extended hospital stay and a quick recovery. So I called in sick on a Friday and my mom (who was an invaluable support system for me at this time) and I met him at the hospital and had the procedure done. I took it easy on Saturday and Sunday and by Monday I was back at work, with a follow-up visit with Dr. Joe scheduled soon after. He mentioned that in the event that we didn't get the entire pregnancy, there was a "day after" pill that I could take that would rid my body of the remainder of the pregnancy.

I woke up on Monday not really feeling very well, but I had my follow up appointment which revealed no issues or complications and went back to work. However, by the time I returned to work I called my mom to tell her that I was in a lot pain. [What's funny about this, and how God works in strange ways… is that at this job everyone always had Advil or Tylenol—this was the music industry and we were always going out; but for some reason, no one on my entire floor had anything that day.] My mom immediately sensed something was wrong and she called Dr. Joe demanding my blood results ASAP.

He called her back soon after and instructed her to get me to the emergency room STAT since I was bleeding internally! Apparently, the pregnancy was in other tube that had not been operated on. The sonogram was apparently not entirely fool proof since it was difficult to distinguish between a blood clot which is what he had removed and the undeveloped fetus. Only the blood test could confirm if the pregnancy had been terminated successfully. My pregnancy had developed too far and had ruptured within my tube. Fortunately for me, my tube had not ruptured completely and caused my immediate death, due a hole the size of a pin in my tube that allowed blood to drip into my body for the past two weeks. To make a long story short, by the end of this process two pints of blood had been drained from my body and three of my major organs; stomach, liver and pancreas had ceased to function correctly. I ended up being on disability leave for five weeks in debilitating pain and in the end, had to have both of my fallopian tubes removed, thus making it 100% certain that if I were to ever become pregnant in the future it would have to be through In Vitro Fertilization.

Whew....so there you have it, my background to IVF in a nutshell. Now the really interesting part of my tale is about to begin.

Marty's Thoughts:

I want to commend my beautiful wife for being so brave to share all elements of the journey we underwent to give birth to our beautiful children. Jennifer wanted this to be as complete retelling as possible, so at various junctures I will add my perspective and thoughts about what was taking place.

Jen had been totally honest with me very early on about the complications she would experience with conceiving and giving birth to a child. Not fully grasping the implications I just wrote them off as I thought to myself, "So what. We can just get it done the other way." I was obviously totally in the dark when it came to IVF and I had no knowledge of the complexity of this procedure and potential for failure. Like Jen, I simply assumed that we would have a baby easily and that we would automatically have twins. Boy was I in for the ride of my life and I was essentially clueless about it.

Part One

IVF BEGINS

Cycle One

Becoming a parent is supposed to be an instinctive and natural process, a rite of passage if you will, for every woman willing to take that path; although I am officially starting my second trimester, I have to be honest with you, this still feels surreal to me. I have not let go 100% and allowed myself to feel pure joy and excitement. I still feel the need to protect my emotions and be strong just in case. This is one of the many "aftershocks" of IVF that we aspiring mothers endure, wherein, essentially we are battling too many disappointments coupled with entirely too much information that we don't need and not enough information that we do need! What is IVF exactly? In layman's terms, IVF is the acronym for In Vitro Fertilization, a process of fertilization that manually combines an egg and sperm in a laboratory dish. Once successful fertilization has been achieved, the embryo that results from this process is transferred, which involves physically inserting the embryo into the uterus.

Most women at some point realize that their menstrual cycle is late and they then proceed to take a home pregnancy test. If they obtain a positive result, they will make a doctor's appointment to confirm this result. At that time they are generally already eight sometimes nine weeks pregnant. This is not the case with women undergoing IVF. When we finally get our positive result it usually comes at the expense of having done, oh I'd say around fifteen home pregnancy tests (speaking from personal experience, of course) generally because we are testing too soon after our transfer and then simply because we are in shock and need constant confirmation until our official Beta blood test happens. When we make our appointment with our doctor, a more accurate Beta blood test is administered that does confirm our pregnancy, at which point IVF'ers are only at about 5 weeks pregnant. This then segues into the most excruciatingly nerve-racking first trimester ever, when mothers literally tip toe through every day activities in a state of constant vigilance and concern so that absolutely no chances are taken that can potentially jeopardize the fate of their baby. But I am jumping way ahead of myself here when I should be starting at the beginning of this journey. So, here it goes...

I knew at age 25 that I would never be able to conceive a child without the direct medical intervention of In Vitro Fertilization. This information was relayed to me following an ectopic pregnancy that I experienced that nearly cost me my life but in the end cost me both Fallopian tubes. When I first learned of this complication, I did not fully grasp the full implications, and since starting a family was not exactly on the top of my list, it was not something that I paid close attention to.

Now, fast-forward 13 years and my husband, Marty and I are anxious to get started on our family. I met Marty more than ten years after this occurred, when I was about 36 years old. By that time, I had of course survived a series of failed relationships and reached a point where I was mentally ready to settle down. We met through his cousin Marc who was a friend of mine and our relationship progressed pretty quickly with us moving in together after six months and becoming engaged at the end of our first year together. At that point we were both ready emotionally to have kids, and being the kind of person who has always worn my heart on my sleeve about everything in my life, I had been open and honest with him and his family from the beginning about the complications inherent with any endeavor on my part to conceive a child. Marty and I married on May 25th 2007, and we actually started the IVF process literally the moment we returned from our honeymoon. Fortunately for us, we were both mature enough and in a great place financially with our career paths and incomes to undertake this process.

I had started preparing for this process a few months earlier by selecting a clinic and having our consultation as well as any and all testing to determine our eligibility taken care of before our wedding. We chose to use a clinic, which was recommended to me by a very close friend who had conceived her beautiful twins there a little over eleven years before, when they were considered the premiere IVF clinic in New York State. We had our consult and we were told that based on my history and the results of subsequent testing by the clinic that I was a great candidate and that I should not experience any problems conceiving through IVF. Although we were fortunate to be in a great position financially to undertake this process, we received fantastic news that my insurance would cover the procedure 100%, so there would be no money out-of-pocket expenses at all. I remember being so euphoric at this stage, relieved that despite not being able to having kids the conventional way that I had found a viable alternative that was easy enough and free (boy, am I in for a rude awakening!). While on our honeymoon, I started on a protocol that included birth control pills. At that time, being told that everything was fine, I didn't really inquire as to *why* I being directed to take birth control pills, I was just informed that this was part of the protocol and I followed their instructions, never thinking that there were other protocols available that did not involve birth control pills. So for the month prior to starting my first IVF procedure, being a complete stickler for the rules, I took my little white pill at approximately the same time every day. That was in May.

June arrives and we have returned from our honeymoon. Marty is out of state in Saratoga, NY working on a great paying show opportunity, and I am in Queens, NY starting the first part of the cycle called the Micro Flare. With Marty out of state, it is a bit rough emotionally, however, I did have a support team in place that was able to inject me in his absence. We have all of our meds, needles and I even have a designated "shoot-up" area. I remember injecting myself for the first time in front of Marty and taking a good five minutes before I could actually "stab" the needle into my stomach "pouch" that I had developed over the past two years. Luckily, I did have people a short drive away in Westchester County and the Bronx willing to inject me when I got too squeamish. It didn't hurt though, these were the easy ones, and although I did bruise easily, strangely enough I was utterly happy. I do not recall being this happy ever, and I took it as a sign that everything in the universe was in perfect alignment and that my successful pregnancy with twins was predestined. It was funny that when I found out that I would need IVF and that multiple births are very common through this process, I imprinted this clear picture in my mind that I would have twins when I conceived, a boy and a girl to be exact.

At this stage I was undergoing the "stim" process, whereby I was injecting Gonal F, Lupron and Menopur in the morning and afternoon at the same time each day at different dosage levels. When you are "stimming" as we IVF'ers call it, you are actually controlling your entire reproductive system. You are dictating your ovulation cycle and producing a significantly larger number of Follicles than you would generate normally in order to produce more eggs. During this phase, which can last approximately 10 – 14 days, every woman is different; you initially go to the office every other day and then every day to have your blood tested (which with my vein less arms is no easy task, I got butchered a couple of times!) and an Ultrasound performed so that the doctors can monitor your follicle growth. This is crucial. The blood checks your Estrogen and Progesterone levels and the Ultrasound makes sure that you have enough Follicles that are growing. Every clinic is different but most have a designated time for these tests to occur which are usually in the morning between the hours of 7-9am on a first-come, first-served basis. I referred to these meetings as the "cattle call" because I saw so many women of every age, color, race and religion in one room all going through the process of trying to make babies! Now, in a way I found this to be reassuring, since clearly I was not the only one in this position, I was also quite impressed with the system that the clinic had in place and how quickly, relatively speaking, you were in and out. First you signed in, and then you were called for blood; you went back to the waiting room and shortly thereafter you were called for your Ultrasound. Then you left. Each afternoon a nurse would call you with your instructions for that evening. The instructions consisted of maintaining the current dosages or increasing/decreasing it as needed. That was my life for approximately 2 weeks and it is all consuming.

TRIGGER HAPPY

With the stim process complete, the HCG injection is the next step in an IVF treatment and is used for triggering the oocytes to go through the last stage of maturation, before they can be retrieved and the timing of this shot is vital. (hCG: human chorionic gonadotropin (hCG) is a hormone produced during pregnancy that is made by the developing placenta after conception). Marty was still in Saratoga, so a friend of mine in Westchester gave me the enormous HCG Trigger shot which means in 36 hours they will retrieve my eggs and Marty will drive down from Saratoga and provide his semen for fertilization.

If the injection is given too early, the eggs would not have matured enough, and if the shot is given too late, the eggs may be "too old" and won't fertilize properly. The daily ultrasounds I started getting right before this shot, were meant to assist the doctors in timing this trigger shot just right. Usually, the injection is given when at least four or more follicles have grown to be 18 to 20mm in size and your estradiol levels are greater than 2,000pg/ML. This shot is a one-time/per cycle injection (yeah!)

Here's the bad part…if as you're approaching the HCG stage, and it's become clear that not enough follicles have grown or if you're at risk for severe ovarian hyper stimulation syndrome, your treatment cycle may be canceled and the shot will not be given at all. If treatment is canceled because your ovaries didn't respond well to that particular selection of medications, your doctor may recommend different medications to be tried on the next cycle. Which means you are back to square one and you have to start and pay for the process all over again.......

(TID BIT: Cancellation happens in 10 to 20% of IVF treatment cycles. The chance of cancellation rises with age, with women older than age 35 more likely to experience treatment cancellations).

About 36 hours after I received the HCG injection (3 days is generally the timing), the egg retrieval took place. Marty drove down from Saratoga and met me on Madison Avenue to provide his sperm. Unfortunately, he couldn't stay for the entire procedure and had to head back soon after, a fact that he felt completely guilt ridden about. I tried to allay his guilt and put his mind at ease, because I felt so confident that my becoming impregnated in this cycle was a virtual certainty. Before the retrieval, an anesthesiologist administered a drug intravenously which helped me to feel relaxed and pain free, and I essentially slept through the entire procedure.

Once the medications took effect, the doctor used what they call a transvaginal ultrasound to guide a needle through the back wall of my vagina and up to my ovaries. He then used the needle to gently suck the fluid and oocyte (egg) from the follicle into the needle. There is one oocyte per follicle. My oocytes were then transferred to the embryology lab for fertilization.

The number of oocytes definitely varies but will generally be guesstimated before the retrieval via ultrasound. (TID BIT: the average number of oocytes is 8 to 15, with more than 95% of patients having at least one oocyte retrieved). In my case I was informed that nine oocytes were retrieved. Since I am not fully aware of what is considered a good number of eggs to have retrieved and since I am thinking that all 9 would fertilize and I could transfer five and freeze four ....well, 9 eggs sounds amazing to me! After a bit longer, they release me and I have a man-size breakfast. The hard part I know is now behind me.

Marty's Thoughts:

Saratoga is about a 3 1/2 hour drive from NYC. I went on tour with the New York City Ballet knowing full well that I would have to drive back down to the city, do my business, and then drive back upstate. There were certain days out of my 2 weeks that would have been more convenient for me to come in for this procedure, but the Saturday morning when it was scheduled was probably the worst day of the week since I absolutely 100% could not miss the matinee performance that day. So I drove down in the middle of the night, arrived at the clinic before they opened and waited in a hallway for signs of life as my clock kept ticking down. When the staff arrived, I completed my part of the deal and prepared to bolt out of there and head back upstate. Just as the elevator door opened Jen stepped out. We hugged for a moment, then soon after I was doing 85 on the thruway and got back to Saratoga with an hour to spare. That moment, by the elevator, is truly one of the top guilt ridden moments of my life.

The Wait

Thinking that the hardest part was behind me was a grave mistake. With all of the shots and retrieval process behind me, I now had 2-4 days not delineated by injections, appointments or anything to do with IVF and I celebrated. I went to the beach with my girlfriend and had some delicious wine. Then the call came. I was not fully aware of the implications of the call that comes the day after the retrieval, but I soon got a rude awakening. This first call informed me of how many of the nine eggs retrieved were actually fertilized. It was at this point that I learned that although nine eggs were retrieved this is no guarantee that all of them will actually fertilize. My first call relayed that only four of the nine fertilized – the first chink to develop in my master plan. Further, I was informed that there was also no guarantee that all of these four fertilized eggs would make it to the transfer scheduled for three days hence. Obviously, quite significant information that in a moment can plummet your euphoric attitude and inject doubt and jitters when you least need it. Reality intruded quite rudely into my dreamlike vision of what this entire process would be. But I struggled to maintain my optimism and thought that although I may not be able to freeze any eggs, surely, out of the four that they transfer at least two will implant and provide me with my instant family. I completed the second component of the call which was to schedule the day three transfer. I then called Marty to relay the news, and went to the beach and drank wine.

T-Day

What a glorious summer morning. Today is the day the Marty and I will conceive our children and this will be the start of our beautiful family. My in-laws will be over the moon, and the entire universe will be informed in a matter of seconds—courtesy of my mother-in-law. My grandparents will have the opportunity to see their only granddaughter present them with two beautiful great-grandchildren. The planets are perfectly aligned, I'm floating on air. It's a perfect day. I arrive at the clinic with my water bottle in-hand as a full bladder is required for the transfer procedure. The initial protocol is very much like the retrieval. I get a key to a locker and I go into a room to change into a robe, lockup my clothes and wait in a small, single-patient waiting room. A short while later, although even 10 minutes is an eternity today, a doctor comes in and tells me that out of the four eggs retrieved, three were genetically bad and I am left with only one to transfer. He goes on to tell me that the one that's left is really a beautiful embryo, grade A, 8-cell, which apparently is very good. However, my only thought at this moment is what???? And what does genetically bad mean??? And why are you dumping this on me NOW right before the transfer when I should be happy & relaxed!! In that moment I am completely deflated, miserable, tortured and alone as Marty is still in Saratoga Springs working with the ballet. The show must go on however, so I head into the same room that I had my retrieval in and with an over-full bladder along with a catheter (I quickly learned how much water is actually necessary to achieve full bladder status) and the procedure is done. I am wheeled back into recovery, fully aware and completely uncomfortable because I have to pee like a race horse and I can't for 20 minutes. So I lay there and the pain in my bladder grows so fierce that I am pushed to peeing in a pan placed underneath me. Not my finest moment especially considering the pee is going everywhere but in the pan! Finally, my time is up and I can go into the bathroom, clean up and leave; my head hung low, the tears streaming down my face, my cell phone in hand ready to call Marty. And all I can think is how did this day get so messed-up?

My husband, Marty is a laid back, "take it in stride" kind of guy, and like most guys, doesn't really wear his emotions on his sleeve. I of course have been feeling that I am doing most of "heavy lifting" during this process, namely, the shots, injections, retrieval, transfer, etc. and he has taken more of a "passenger seat" in this. Obviously, with so many hormones traversing my body and my emotional struggle with this entire process, he has had to deal with my mood swings and he has been treading very lightly these days. As soon as I exit the building, I lean up against the wall and call him crying. As hopeful as I am, I am also a realist and I know full well that at my age the odds of this one embryo implanting are slim. I am also so discouraged because for as long as I have known that I would need IVF, I wanted twins. I can tell Marty is disappointed and sad that he can't be here for this. So now we wait the two weeks and to see what happens…

THE TWO-WEEK WAIT...

I may only be speaking for myself on this point, but the idea behind doing IVF and enduring all the injections, the appointments, the constant retrieval of blood, the rotation of doctors prodding you for the ultrasound, and of course the agonizing wait that you are about to endure is to have more than one egg placed back inside you. I mean seriously, my body already produces one friggin' egg a month! So here it goes the real excruciating wait. I have to mention that during this time, during this entre journey really, but specifically during this time, my friends Gigi and Gina are on stand-by for me in case I need to talk or vent. During this interminable two week wait I call them constantly… At first, I'm not optimistic; this just isn't how I thought any of this would play out. Even when I was 25 and I knew my reproductive situation, I thought that I would have twins; the "instant family"-and that would be that! Each day that passes is worse than the prior and the thoughts that run through my head are exhausting. I have always been a fan of rationalization; it's what has gotten me through a slew of mistakes and "mishaps" in my life. However, the amount of rationalization that I am applying now is mind boggling. I am twisting and turning every twinge, every bit of slight soreness into a pregnancy.

I had a strong support network at this time from my husband, immediate and extended family and friends. Everyone is very supportive, and of course because I am telling everyone everything, they are as let down and disappointed as I am, but let's face it...almost everyone on my side and on Marty's side have no idea what IVF really is, and even when I try to explain it they really don't get it. Then there are the other folks and honestly I don't know who they are but they exist on both sides of our family who are still wondering why I can't just have kids the "normal" way and what did I do to find myself in this situation. So while you are going through all of this and you do have support you are wondering what people are really thinking and you're wondering what if this doesn't work...how everyone will feel then. At least I felt that way and no matter how many times Marty told that he married me for me, I still felt this enormous amount of pressure and isolation because I felt that no one could truly grasp what I was feeling.

It is also at this time that I discovered a truly amazing website www.ivf-infertility.com which I believe is based in the UK but is as global a site as I have ever come across. There are tons of IVF sites out there but hands down (in my opinion) this is the most comprehensive, easily navigated site with TONS of information on every aspect of infertility. It doesn't take long for me to find the latest "2WW" (2 week wait) posting and dive right in. There are so many women who are going through the exact same thing that I am at the very same moment; it is reassuring in a twisted sort of way. I began to read each woman's story, and the stories are all so very different and the reasons for infertility run the gamut from female tubular problems to unexplained male morphology issues. I am learning so much, and I am already hearing about different protocols that each doctor/clinic uses. In some respect there is so much information that it verges into the realm of information overload that makes me question the very process that I had just undergone.

I register my login and password, which is not clever or baby longing as some I come across, such as "waiting to be a mommy," I just use the name I always use, for every site I register on. I quickly learn what all of the acronyms stand for, for example: DH (Dear Husband), PMA (Positive Mental Attitude) and my personal favorite POAS (Pee on a Stick), and I create my first posting. I swear I think this site is largely what got me through the 2WW without completely losing my mind. Every day I post what new symptoms I am feeling, looking for validation that I am in fact pregnant. The one symptom that I seem to come across a lot that seems connected with a BFP (Big Fat Positive) is cramping during the 2WW. Some of what I read ranges from slight cramping to excruciating pain for a small amount of time. Women on the board will say that cramping is an excellent sign that your little embies are in fact implanting, and that is what causing the cramping. However, there is a couple of "experts" on the site and none of them will confirm a direct correlation between cramping and implantation leading to a BFP. Needless to say, I experienced no cramping at all.

The days go by slowly and I am finally at day 6 of my 12 day wait before my Beta Blood test, when I decide that I will POAS. By this time, Marty is home and we have been enduring the wait together. He is very much against me taking the pregnancy test so early but at this point his feelings cannot deter me from going ahead with the premature test. Now mind you, day 6 is too early to test especially with just one embryo transferred. But that doesn't stop me. Of course, the test comes back negative, I am devastated but I proceed to pee on five more sticks in quick succession! All negative. I post my dismal results on the site and everyone's response is the same; I can absolutely be pregnant with a low Beta and over-the-counter pregnancy tests need a certain Beta number in order to be detected. Okay, I muster up a bit of optimism.

Finally, my two week wait elapses and it is the morning of my Beta test. I go to the office; they take my blood and tell me that they will call me between 1-4pm. This has got to be the longest day of my life. Finally, at 2:12pm the phone rings and I can immediately tell by the Nurse's tone of voice that I am not pregnant. She apologizes and we hang up. I am hysterical and I call Marty. Then I go to the liquor store and I buy a BIG bottle of white wine. I proceed to get drunk and call my girlfriends. I allow myself to get nice and drunk and wallow in self-pity however I don't allow myself to stay in that "neighborhood" for very long because the longer you stay there the harder it is to get back on track. I am not IVF jaded yet nor am I completely disillusioned. We will take our follow-up meeting with Dr. G and we will try again! This is just a small bump in the road. Marty and I are disappointed but we are certain the number two is our time!

Marty's Thoughts:

Receiving this phone call from Jen that day added to my feeling of overwhelming guilt. Here I was, back in Saratoga on my day off, happy and content thinking twins were about to grow in my wife's belly. Taking that call and listening to my wife cry killed me. I should have been with her. What kind of man is not there to hold his wife in his arms and provide direct, physical comfort to his wife on such a traumatic day of her life? What kind of fool am I really? All of these questions were running through my brain at a rapid pace. This was devastating for me as well but I knew that Jen took this especially hard. Little did I know, but this was the 1st of many let downs to come.

On the Road to Number Two

We take our meeting with Dr. G and he basically tells me that the qualities of my embryos are less than great quality. This has been determined by my high FSH number (Follicle Secreting Hormone) which was 16.8. This is the first that I am hearing of a FSH number and I am now provided with a full explanation about why I was placed on birth control pills the month prior to starting the procedure. Apparently the pill can lower your FSH. In layman's terms, higher the FSH number, the worse your embryo quality. At this clinic any number lower than a 12 is considered fine, and obviously the lower number the better.

I quickly learn that I need to educate myself on the process because the doctors simply do not tell you all of the minute details of the IVF process. You need to ask a ton of questions and do independent research.

At the end of our meeting it was determined that we will use the "Antagonist" protocol for the upcoming second cycle. The Antagonist protocol utilizes injectable drugs called Cetrotide and Antagon to prevent premature ovulation. Lupron which I had used in this first cycle has short lived stimulatory effects while antagonists shut down the pituitary gland immediately.

This antagonist protocol is generally used for women who are donating eggs and for women not producing good quality eggs. This protocol is also more aggressive in assisting your ovaries in producing better quality eggs.

Cycle Two

I don't want to be stuck in a morass of negativity and I am certainly not entertaining any thoughts of giving up on our commitment to creating additions to the Prudenti family, so I immediately embark upon cycle two, a few short months after our unsuccessful cycle one. I feel that having gone through the process before, I am now armed with hard earned knowledge of what to expect and how to temper my expectations.

It is now October 2007, and we begin cycle two. Marty is home for this, and having someone with a direct appreciation for what I was experiencing, made it easier for me. I felt really good about it. It's just a second cycle, no big deal. The shots are the same, and already I feel like a pro. As far as details of this cycle go, it is pretty much the same length of time and the exact monitoring procedures. This time as the Retrieval day approaches I am less exuberant and more cautiously optimistic. I am armed with more knowledge this time around. At the Retrieval, Marty is with me and they announce that they retrieved 15 eggs!! This is obviously fantastic news for us, especially in light of the fact that for the last cycle that number was nine eggs... We are very happy. Of course, we must endure the three day wait, so we repress our happiness and we wait.

I am at work when I receive the call announcing that 12 eggs had been fertilized. Wow! This cycle is looking like it's going to be the one that produces the Prudenti clan! Of course, as I do with every bit of good news I proceed to make the rounds of calls to Marty, and my invaluable circle of support; my mother-in-law and my network of girlfriends. Each one of them highly invested in this journey with me and there for me 100%.

T-Day Take Two

Marty was home to administer the HCG trigger shot (no added stress of trying to find someone to inject me in the buttocks) and 36 hours later we find ourselves in the same room again. The only important difference is that this time Marty is there for me through the entire the transfer process. As I did the last time, I go into the room, change and wait in another room for the doctor to come in and tell us how many eggs they are transferring. We are very hopeful. With the larger number of fertilized eggs we hope that we can transfer more than the one egg we had for the previous cycle.

At the clinic, the facility is set-up where there are about 3 to 4 rooms side by side filled with waiting couples. It is therefore entirely possible to hear what the doctor is saying to the couple ahead of you through the paper thin walls, and we managed to hear what the doctor says to the couple before us—they are having five eggs transferred! WOW!

The doctor walks into our room and tells us that we have three beautiful, grade A, 8 cell, no fragments embryos that they are going to transfer. In this heady moment of excitement I can tell you that certain questions that I wanted to ask and points I wanted to raise with the doctor were the furthest things from my mind, as I was so caught up in the emotions of the moment. Thankfully, Marty was with me and he had no qualms stating that we had overheard the doctor informing the couple next door of their five eggs being transferred and asking for an explanation of why we were only having three eggs transferred. The doctor goes on to explain that this is their 3rd attempt, they are older than us and frankly the qualities of their eggs are not as "good" as ours. All valid answers, I suppose and we had no reason to question him. In the end, they transfer three and we did get so caught up in the moment that we forgot to ask how many were being frozen for later use!

In the end, we leave there happy. We have three gorgeous embryos in my body right now! Three! Seriously, one out of these three is going to implant, right? Of course - cautious optimism is thrown to the wind at this juncture.

ENTER 2WW—AGAIN!

Thank God for IVF-infertility.com. I swear this site alone saved my sanity, simply because this medium lets you know that you are not alone and that there are many others going through exactly what you are. It provides a judgment free forum where you can share every crazy thought that runs through your "bad neighborhood" of a head that you are afraid to share with your family and friends lest they think you crazy, or they are just tired of hearing from you yet again. Your fellow posters provide that support, reassurance and invaluable insight from past experiences that I cannot get anywhere else. I post every day, several times a day! Once again, most of the symptoms that leads a lot of the women on the boards to BFP's, I do not experience. I hold out a little longer than I did in cycle one and have not taken a home pregnancy test yet, so I remain cautiously optimistic—until day 7.

Day 7—not pregnant and so begins the obsessive need to test every day until my Beta. I'll cut to the chase on this one. Every day leading up to my Beta the tests are negative and on the day of my Beta I get my period. Needless to say, we are faced with another no pregnancy.

Two weeks later, we meet with Dr. G who now suggests that we use donor eggs, something that we had hoped would never become a consideration. We were therefore at a crossroad. We can stay with the current clinic and initiate another cycle which they will oversee if we insist, but we know that at this point they are not very supportive of the idea nor are they at all confident of success. I can certainly appreciate their concerns since our failure to conceive especially with the onset of a new cycle would only lower their success rates, which is not good for an industry wherein infertility clinics literally are defined by their rates of successful conceptions.

I do know that I am not ready to use someone else's eggs and I know that Marty is not into that idea at all. In fact, he would prefer to stop trying altogether if the only option is to use someone else's embryos. So we thank Dr. G for everything they have done for us and we leave with the intention of going to another clinic and trying again. Having no intention of abandoning my quest to have children, I also start the process of researching the world of donor eggs, just as a plan B.

Marty's Thoughts:

During this second cycle, I'm home from Saratoga and I have to do the one thing I have been dreading for this process, sticking my wife in the backside with a 1 ½ inch long needle. The drug was called progesterone, an oil based fluid that took forever to ooze out of the syringe. The first time I administered this injection it took me 10 minutes before I actually stabbed Jen with the needle. As time went on, I would become a pro at this. At this time, I would also talk to the one embryo in Jen's belly and say things like, "I believe in you" and "please stick". Therefore this second phone call delivering the disappointment news that the procedure was unsuccessful was especially devastating. I remember looking at Jen and saying "we could stop the shots now."

What was even more demoralizing was that although Jen's insurance covered in full our first attempt, we had no such coverage *for this cycle from her insurance or mine. Therefore, we had to delve into our savings to the extent of $20, 000 when all was said and done.*

I was also very much against the idea of donor eggs even though I knew that I was being selfish about this, but I just couldn't embrace the idea. Another thing that irked me was the fact that Dr. G wrote us off with his negativity. This prompted us to look for other doctors. I harbored a lot of resentment for that clinic after that day.

Mid-Point Breakdown

Let me just preface this point of the story by stating that I have been through a lot of life altering stuff in my 38 years on this planet. But that is an autobiography of its own!

Okay, so relatively speaking I remain semi-positive, not entirely losing my mind in front of people, but I am in a bad place right now! There has never been a point in my life when I did not want children or thought I would not have children—never, ever a moment. Now I am faced with a brand new reality that I am not remotely mentally or emotionally equipped to handle. Added to this, is the fact that I feel this silent but unrelenting pressure (completely self-imposed) about creating new titles for my in-laws. As it stands right now, as the newlyweds, it's up to me to make them grandparents. Up to me! I don't think that anyone can truly grasp the degree of anxiety that conjures up within me. Marty has been beyond supportive throughout this entire process. He assured me that if it wasn't meant for us to have kids then we won't and that he will be happy with just the two of us, since I am all the family he wanted when we got married (not to mention our cat Jezebel and new kitten, Smudge). Sure he wants kids but he did not marry me for me to produce kids for him. He married me because I am the woman that he wants to spend the rest of his life with.

Of course hearing this is wonderful and it does help a little, but it is almost impossible to believe in his words 100%, and honestly it didn't matter what he said because I was destined to have babies. I truly believed that if we weren't able to have a family it would adversely affect our marriage because I would always feel inadequate and incomplete as a woman and wife. I am 100% certain of this and I am honest about how I feel with him as well as my mother-in-law. I am very fortunate to have a very supportive mother-in-law who is a wreck because I am wreck and who knows that although Marty may not verbalize his feelings, he's a wreck too. So, as you can see, I am indeed in a bad place right now, still reeling from the implications of this latest failure as well as my feelings of responsibility for my husband's and mother-in-law's disappointment.

So I wallow in self-pity and too much wine (again) for a few weeks, but then I decide that the next place for us will be CRMI - Center for Reproductive Medicine and Fertility. I go online, do my research and find out that CRMI and New York Presbyterian are tied as the top fertility clinics in New York. I couldn't let too much time elapse where self-doubt would set in. A huge part of getting through this is barreling on completely focused on the end goal. In fact you need to assume the mantle of a warrior forging ahead despite any temporary setback and not allowing time for your emotions or pain to get the best of you. Although, I will admit, they did a pretty good job on me this time around.

It is now the end of October or early November and I call CRMI to set-up a consultation with Dr. R., the head Doctor at CRMI, but I am informed that he is not available for a consultation for at least a couple of months, so on the recommendation of the nurse handling the call I decide to go with Dr. C., who also happens to head up the donor egg program at CRMI. Marty and I have our consultation with Dr. C. and I bring her all my records that I had requested from the last clinic. We have what seems to be a great, 2 ½ hour consultation. She is very thorough and makes us feel that she is genuinely appreciative of our overriding desire to start a family and empathetic of our past experience with IVF. At the end of the consultation, she does suggest that I obtain my medical records from my gynecologist so that she can have a better understanding of my medical history that made IVF mandatory for me. My recollection so many years after the fact is a bit fuzzy and she'd like to have complete clarity of my particular medical background, which makes total sense.

Funny how such a mundane request launched us onto a new path and what is one of the most important twists in our story. I reach out to my old OB/GYN, Dr. F., who had been my Gynecologist from the age of 18 until about 27 or so. He saved my life when I had an ectopic pregnancy that ruptured causing internal hemorrhaging (I told you that I had been through some life-altering stuff, and that was just the tip of the iceberg!). I had no desire to switch doctors, but he had stopped accepting my insurance and his fees were too expensive for me to pay out-of-pocket at that time in my life. I successfully reconnected with him and I brought him up to speed on my situation and filled him in on my most recent consultation at CRMI. He immediately recommends that I see a colleague of his - Dr. K. for no other reason than he knows him and respects his work immensely. He also suggested that Dr. K.'s personality was a great complement to mine and he felt that we would work well together. Now, while I may not have spoken to Dr. F. in over ten years, this is a man that I HGHLY RESPCT and he had an unblemished history with me and my mother. My mother loved him. So when he spoke, I just listened and I trusted him.

I immediately called Dr. K.'s office and explain my situation to his assistant mentioning that I just spoken to Dr. F., and just like that I have a new consult appointment and I am informed that I don't need to follow-up with Dr. C.; they will do that for me. Now the events that follow I am going to mention because I was completely flabbergasted by the entire situation. No sooner had I hung up the phone with Dr. K.'s office than I receive a call from Dr. C.'s office asking me why I was switching? I briefly explain why and assume that this was the end of it, but it's not and this process starts becoming needlessly stressful. Dr. C.'s office refuses to release my records or to release me as a patient, it is beyond absurd. I find myself in the uncomfortable position of calling back and forth between both offices trying to figure out what is going on…finally the piece de resistance… Dr. C. calls me and asks me why I have decided to switch to Dr. K. Really? Are you kidding me? I am approaching my third IVF procedure and I am being confronted and stressed out about my choice in doctors after ONE consultation? Dr. C. then takes this debacle a step further and calls Dr. F. asking him why he does not like her?? Needless to say I laid into her and it was resolved. Clearly she had no idea who she had messed with.

We finally have our consultation with Dr. K. in November and we love him! He had already spoken with Dr. F., who had brought him up to speed on my medical history, but there were a few facts that even Dr. F. was fuzzy on, given how long ago my ectopic pregnancy had occurred. Dr. K. goes over the medical protocol for this cycle and decides that the first thing he wants to do is a Hysteroscopy, that is, the inspection of the uterine cavity by endoscopy with access through the cervix. Essentially, he uses a thin telescope that is inserted through the cervix into the uterus. The point of this procedure is to observe the endometrial cavity (inside of the uterus) and make sure my remaining tubes are not causing any trouble. The result of this procedure indicates that all is fine. Dr. K. then conducts another procedure called co-culture which is very interesting. The basic concept involves growing embryos in a culture medium on top of a layer of cells such as fallopian tube cells or cells from the lining of the uterus called endometrial cells (in my case the latter). The idea is that these cells will stimulate development of the embryos by removing toxins from the medium, adding growth factors, and possibly aiding in implantation through familiarity. This procedure takes only 3-5 minutes BUT I found it to be quite painful. They also take about 6 huge vials of blood twice for this procedure (before you start stimming and afterwards) and getting that much blood from me is very challenging. I also went on birth control pills the month prior to my cycle. So when this is all completed I was ready for stimming in January. It will be a new year, a new IVF clinic—I am feeling renewed and totally positive. This is it!

Third Time's a Charm

It's time to start my third and hopefully successful cycle, and at this juncture I should mention that we are pretty much down to using the rest of our savings for this particular cycle as insurance coverage is pretty much nil at this juncture. The protocol from this point on is the same as cycle two with the added assistance of the Co-Culture procedure. The set-up at CRMI is also pretty much identical to the last clinic, in that you go in for monitoring from 7-9am and they take blood and then you get called again for the Ultrasound. The wait isn't that bad and luckily I am working on the East side at 46th and Third and CRMI is located at 68th and York so the commute back and forth isn't too bad. I have to mention and give kudos to my husband, who drove me in every time I had monitoring done, which was extremely helpful. I also have to mention the next thing that gets introduced into this cycle, which in the end I believe proved to be invaluable - the introduction of an Acupuncturist! I begin to see Aimee Raupp who had actually been recommended me to me some time ago, even before I had started IVF, as someone who could help with the knots in my shoulders and neck.

I had never called her. However, when I started a new job at W Magazine, my boss and friend mentions her again and swears by her. I subsequently called Aimee and it turned out that she specialized in infertility challenges. We met and immediately established a great connection. She asked a lot of questions about my particular situation and I provided her with detailed information about my fibroid and the challenges that I have been experiencing with conceiving. Aimee was so obviously cognizant about the subject of infertility as well as the intricacies of the various IVF procedures that I felt completely comfortable with her.

During the month when I was taking birth control pills but before I started stimming, I actually had about 4 sessions with Aimee. Although she had assured me that Acupuncture during stimming was perfectly fine, I was too skittish and I appreciated the fact that she supported that decision. My stimming went off without a hitch and my follicles grew modestly but well. At the end of the day I believe I had 12 follicles and it was time to trigger!

T-Day Take Three (Really??)

I can't believe this is our third go around. They say third time's a charm, right? I hold fast to this saying, although for every cycle I had undergone so far I had felt that it was the one! But this one had to be successful, especially since we had incorporated new procedures and I had started seeing Aimee. Marty once again administered the HCG injection and 36 hours later we are ready for the retrieval.

Turns out that we have nine embryos! Fantastic! Of course, we know that we now have to wait until three days later when I have my transfer done to find out how many actually fertilized. Fast forward three days… we have five embryos and they are transferring four. Once again, they are all gorgeous grade A embryos that are: 8, 7, 7, 6 cells! We have no qualms or questions and are very happy with the transfer of the four embryos. The one thing that I did differently for this cycle was that I went for a one hour acupuncture session before and after the transfer for one hour.

Now I have four embryos in my body… how can I possibly not be pregnant this time?

Do I Even Need To Title This?

Did I mention how IVF-infertility.com saved my sanity? I lived on this site. What's interesting and different about this 2WW is that twice during the wait you report to CRMI for a blood test. The blood tests your Estrogen levels. I actually didn't ask any questions about this test at all. I just went in, took it and that was that! Of course you know that at the 7 day mark I took a pregnancy test and it was negative. I will save you all the suspense on this one... we are not pregnant. What stinks is that you know the second you hear the nurse's voice on the other end of the phone. She does not want to call you and tell you this at all. Dr. K. also called me, which I thought was very nice and we actually scheduled our follow-up at that moment.

That evening we had plans to go out to dinner with Marty's parents and we decided not to cancel. I didn't want any quiet time to sit down and obsess over this latest setback. That didn't stop me from trying to dampen my pain with some wine before we left for dinner as well as more wine when we arrived. I of course didn't have much of an appetite, so you get where this is going, right? It gets better. On the way home, fortunately in MY car, I proceed to throw up at the window. Luckily I was drinking white wine and lucky for Marty and his mom, who got stuck cleaning up after me, I had no food in my stomach so it was not that big of a mess at all. The next day I woke up hung over, depressed and embarrassed.

Beyond Breakdown

Where do I begin? First of all, we have no money left in our savings. Secondly, I am completely disheartened and I'm forced to face the stark reality that I may not be able to conceive with my eggs at all. I have reached such a state of anxiety that I broach the donor egg scenario to Marty, but he is still not very keen on this prospect, at least not yet anyway. I came to the painful realization that in order to maintain my sanity that I had to step back and not be so consumed by this process anymore. I also felt that my body was stuck in such a "negative space" and that it would be beneficial to take a break and cleanse my body of all of the drugs and hormones and start anew. In addition, since we had completely depleted our funds and did not have the financial wherewithal to start another cycle, I decided before my meeting with Dr. K. that I would take a 6 month break.

Our meeting with Dr. K. goes well. He is very sympathetic to our situation, and reassured us that on paper there is no reason that he can find that would prevent me from conceiving with my own eggs. He does mention that he had noticed that in the two blood tests I had prior to the Beta pregnancy test that my Estrogen level had significantly dropped after the transfer. He knew by day 6 that I was not pregnant because in order to maintain a pregnancy my Estrogen and Progesterone levels needed to be at a certain level. In his opinion I was definitely having an implantation issue which was difficult to account for because doctors simply don't know why some eggs implanted and others don't. I know that at this point Marty has become completely disheartened, and has resigned himself to the fact that maybe us having children was not meant to be. I am emotionally and mentally drained.

My friends and family are completely supportive and a few of my friends are adamant that I don't give up and are quite vocal about their feelings that I am destined to be a mom. I'm not going to give up but right now I just can't invest any more energy into this. I feel as though I have been flying in a "gotta get pregnant" holding pattern for months and months. A pre-programmed robot forging ahead on a mission and not really allowing any emotions in for too long and quite frankly I'm broken and I need to repair myself. I also believe that my body is in a state of "not pregnant" and it needs time to have a few menstrual cycles, get all of the built up hormones out of my system and simply repair itself.

This is in February, and it is at this time that I resume acupuncture with Aimee and based on her recommendation, I begin taking liquid Chinese herbs that are specifically meant to reduce the Fibroid, improve the quality of my eggs and create a friendly reproductive environment for my future babies. This decision was completely personal on my part and I decide that I would not tell Dr. K. about these herbs since I have an intuition that he would not approve. I have absolute trust in Aimee's judgment and decide that I will stop the herbs about 1 ½ months before I even start my 4th cycle. I decided on the liquid version of the herbs because they are the strongest. It tastes like dirt when you drink it, I'm not exaggerating. But surprisingly enough I craved my twice daily, dirt tasting Chinese herbs, and they made me feel great.

Every two weeks without fail I saw Aimee for my Acupuncture treatments. I have never been so committed to anything before in my life. I looked forward to my sessions and rain or shine I was there. I am pretty certain that Marty does not subscribe to these homeopathic or Eastern treatments, but he defers to me and does not voice an opinion. Of course, there's a part of me that feels that if I don't get pregnant he will secretly blame the Acupuncture and herbs, but I felt compelled to include this treatment because I believed in it.

I also have started working out more consistently by incorporating walking into my routine. A friend of mine actually turned me onto Leslie Sansone and all of her Walk for Life DVD's. I do not like gyms or commuting to gyms so this was the perfect workout routine for me.

My general attitude had significantly improved and I feel like both my body and my mind are back in synch. Something is very different about this cycle though. I'm not sure how to explain what I'm feeling except to say that I am just not as consumed with the entire process and emotional baggage inherent with it that permeated all of the previous cycles. I know that probably sounds incomprehensible but I just don't care as much as I did with the prior cycles. Maybe because I've resigned myself to the donor eggs route, I'm not sure. I think that Marty feels the same way as well. One thing that I will say about my feelings is that I am certainly not as stressed out about this cycle.

As we approach the start date in June of the following year, I start my birth control pills again and begin my dialog with the nurses. This protocol will once again be the Antagonist protocol and we will be incorporating the co-culture procedure. He will also put me on an Estrogen patch that I will wear for 24 hours starting Day 3 after the transfer.

Now before I even started the actual cycle I have to mention that a couple of things went wrong that might have indicated to some that this cycle was doomed. The first was regarding the various meds that are required during the cycle. If you are familiar with IVF you know that all the drugs that are needed from start to finish can cost you around $10k. Well, one night when I came home from work and finally made my way to the kitchen to cook dinner, I noticed something. I went to fridge and our butter had melted all over everything and then I noticed that the inside of the fridge was hot! I felt our meds, roughly around $2500 worth, and they were HOT! I could not believe it. I was starting my cycle in one week and I had ruined some of our meds. How did this happen? Well, when I went to shut the fridge door in the morning I didn't slam the door hard enough and the weight of all the condiments in the door panel caused the door to stay ajar about 2 inches all day long! Needless to say, Marty thought it was an idiotic but innocent mistake and we had to charge those meds onto a credit card and rush delivery. The second incident, which was pure stupidity on my part, was that I called a psychic who specializes in IVF for a reading. She actually told me that I should not go through with this cycle because I was not going to get pregnant. Normally something like that would completely consume and then break me but this time it rolled right off my back and I started to think, "How can I not be pregnant this time? This time which is our last time with our own eggs…? How can I not be?" Although even with that thought in my head I was still approaching this cycle with the attitude that if it's meant to be it will be—it's in God's hands.

Marty's Thoughts:

This is it. If Jen didn't get pregnant it just wasn't meant to be. Regardless of what she says, under no circumstances would I agree to use donor eggs. I fully recognize how selfish this is, but I cannot accept the fact that Jen would be carrying children who will not be genetically hers. In my perspective she would essentially be a baby carrier only in such a scenario. Dr. K was very honest with us after the 3rd attempt failed. He had that give it one more try attitude and I could tell it had nothing to do with money. We were in a great place now. You could tell something was different about this cycle. Jen swears it was the herbs and her acupuncture sessions, but I say it was fate.

All Our Eggs are Literally in This Basket

Here we go. It's June and I am starting my birth control pills. I am also cutting back on smoking and drinking. My diet has been fine, I am exercising fairly regularly plus I have been on pre-natal vitamins for about a year now! We are still saving as we go and we actually had to charge the IVF meds and my Chinese herbs, which incidentally were $250 a cycle. Towards the end of birth control month I go into the office for my blood test to check my FSH levels and to give the six vials of blood that are needed for the co-culture procedure. I also have the co-culture procedure performed.

As July approaches, I allow myself some leeway to drink at our Cousin Gina's wedding. Gina's wedding is held at Giando on the Water in Brooklyn where Marty and I got married. The owner is Marty's uncle and Gina's dad, what a wedding it was and boy did I drink. The last time I drank was I believe, June 12th (not 100% sure) and it was at a Melissa Etheridge concert. Shortly after that I began taking my stimming meds. Just like the prior three cycles I reported for blood and US every other day and the progress was modest but steady. In the end I ended up with 12 follicles, which seems to be the norm for me. Of those 12, nine fertilized, again no big surprise there.

I did fit in an acupuncture session before my procedure on transfer day, but did not go post transfer simply because I didn't want to drive unnecessarily on New York City streets. When we arrive we were told that seven embryos fertilized and they would transfer five, which is wonderful. For the record, we insisted CRMI transfer the absolute maximum number of embryos and we would sign any necessary documents that allowed them to do so. We didn't have to sign anything and given my past record with IVF they felt comfortable transferring five. Dr. K. felt very optimistic about this cycle and went as far as to say that this was the cycle! As far the other two embryos, they told us that they would watch them. In all honesty I didn't even give those two eggs much thought after the transfer day.

Once we get back home I am in bed and relaxing for the next two days. Once I go back to work I just take my commute which involves the railroad, two subways and walking a total of about 15 blocks very leisurely. Two days after my transfer I begin using the Estrogen patch which stays on me 24 hours a day and gets changed every other day. My first blood test will be on Day 4. The wait begins...

I'd say that around day three while I am asleep I'm awakened by pretty painful cramps. Glorious cramps! I immediately wake up Marty to tell him that I have cramps and he knows that I've never experienced cramping before and of course we take this as a good sign. All the IVF boards that I have read where women have experienced cramping after implantation received BFP (big fat positive) at their Beta. On Day 4 I head into the city for the first of two pre-Beta blood tests that looks at my Estrogen and Progesterone levels and I request that they call me with my results which they won't necessarily do with these two tests unless you request it. It is probably around 3pm when the nurse calls me and I make sure I am around to pick up the phone so that I can pick her brain a little. She tells me my level which I can't recall now and I ask her if this is a good indicator that I may be pregnant. Of course she is not going to put herself that far out on a limb BUT she does say that it is a very good level. So now with a bit more optimism we continue to wait. I know that by day 6 I will be buying a pregnancy test because I just can't help myself. Marty is totally against this and wants no part of it!

On Day 6 I take the second blood test and get the same response from the nurse that calls me with the results. I also bought a pregnancy test the night before so I take that too. It's negative. That's okay it's only Day 6 and I know that is too early. I decide that I'll take another test on Day 8.

On the morning of Day 8 I am planning on driving to PA and spending the weekend with my very best friend Bo who is practically a sister. That morning I take another HPT. This one is not a digital test but the plus and minus sign one. After I take the test and I stare at it for what seems like hours I can swear that I see the faintest vertical line trying desperately to appear. I call Bo in a state of combined shock, euphoria and sheer craziness and tell her that I am bringing the stick for her to see. She can make the determination. Of course she sees it too and insists that I take another one at that very moment. I take a digital one this time and it says pregnant! We are screaming and laughing and generally acting like silly girls. This also begins a weekend of non-stop test taking. In total I take about 15 tests—a combination of digital and plus/minus sign ones. We soon come to realize that the digital tests are easily supplying us with that instant gratification and we want to see the plus sign actually get darker and darker so we opt for more of those. I do call Marty and I tell him. He will not believe anything until our official blood test, but I know inside he is busting a little!

The day of my Beta test is one of the most excruciating days ever and as I soon come to realize one of many excruciating days that I will experience.

Part Two

BUNS IN THE OVEN

Shock. Joy. Surreal.

After taking the test, I return to work where I wait literally on pins and needles for "the call". At 2:13pm my cell phone rings, and I pick up immediately. It is my assigned IVF head nurse, Jeanette. She relays information about my levels to me and confirms that I am indeed pregnant, very pregnant! The hope that I felt after taking the home pregnancy tests can no longer be confined. I am euphoric, I am ecstatic, consumed with a feeling of giddy disbelief, relief and satisfaction that this day is finally here. I hang up the phone and tell the girls at work. Of course we all hug and scream and I am crying with unmitigated joy. These ladies are just as excited if not even more so for me. They had all become personally invested and have been with me throughout my entire journey to this point from the devastating failure of the first cycle through this final triumph. I am then granted the happy opportunity to call Marty and tell him the news, as I know that he too is anxiously awaiting word from me about "the call". I dial his number and he picks up instantly and straight to the point asks "did they call?" I reply "yes" and I can feel his palpable anxiety as he waits for my next words. Eager to put him out of his misery I quickly tell him "Marty, we're pregnant, very pregnant according to my levels." Like me when I heard the news, he is in shock, total disbelief and begins to ask me questions like "are you sure?" and "are you serious?" We quickly decide to conference in his mom who was in the Hamptons at the time. I dial her cell number and Marty does the initial speaking. I can't fully describe and give justice to the ensuing crying and scream fest we engaged in as our family celebrated this momentous news, full of joy, relief and anticipation. I then proceeded to call all of my girlfriends! August 10th became a red letter historic day for us. We are overjoyed, my friends and family are elated for us. Our dreams of having a family are finally coming true. It is so surreal and wonderful and I can't even put into words what we're feeling.

Now begins a new kind of journey. A journey even more nerve wracking than the process of trying to get pregnant—the nine months wait. Buckle up; it's going to be a bumpy ride...

The First 10 Weeks

It is important to understand that women who undergo IVF and are blessed with positive results are receiving this information much earlier than a woman who may take a home pregnancy test after a missed period and receives a positive result. In this instance she is already at least 6 weeks along and then makes an appointment with her Gynecologist for a blood test. We (IVF'ers) are finding out a good 2-4 weeks ahead of time and trust me when I tell you that it makes the journey of getting to three months agonizingly long and torturous.

Once we receive the positive news we quickly schedule an Ultrasound so that the doctor can ensure that he sees the sacs. It will also be at these Ultrasounds that they confirm the number of sacs, thereby determining if we will be having twins or triplets. Two Ultrasounds later, it is confirmed that we are having twins. They then listen for the babies' heartbeat before they release me to my Obstetrician. They do this for about two weeks (one appointment per week) and when they felt that the heartbeats were strong enough, they sign me off and I am on my way.

During one of our Ultrasound appointments, Dr. K. asked me if I had spoken with Dr. F. whom I affectionately call Dr.

Joe about assuming the role as our Obstetrician for the babies. I responded that I hadn't but only due to the fact that Dr. Joe did not participate in our insurance network and we couldn't afford to pay the requisite out-of-pocket expenses of going outside the insurance's network. Dr. K. urges me to reach out despite this because Dr. Joe had expressed a real interest in wanting to deliver our babies. Of course I call Dr. Joe and he very generously accommodates us in such a way that we are able to designate him as our Obstetrician. As we schedule our first appointment with Dr. Joe, everything is falling beautifully into place and we are completely excited to undertake the next steps on our journey.

THE 14TH WEEK CATASTROPHE

I am at work and for all intents and purposes I am healthy and feeling great. I am in the midst of dealing with one of our more "difficult" sales people, when I suddenly feel a rush of fluid gushing from down below. Throughout my pregnancy thus far, I had a discharge to the extent that I wore panty liners every day. Thinking that this was just a regular discharge, albeit a strong one, I did not panic. I got up from my desk and started walking toward the bathroom. As I am doing this I feel fluid running down my leg. Let me back up a bit and inform you that I am wearing a min-dress with tights and a thong underneath. Enough said.

I get to the bathroom, sit down on the toilet and immediately discover that I am bleeding uncontrollably. I am not spotting I am literally a prop in a horror movie with blood gushing out of me. There is a woman in the next stall that overhears my obvious and totally understandable freak out and asks if everything is okay. I tell her that I am three months pregnant with twins and bleeding profusely – can she please walk down the hall and get the girls that I work with. She immediately complies. Thank goodness for the girls. IF this had to happen to me, I am so thankful that it unfolded as it did. The girls come running in, all four of them! I am hysterical. Right away someone calls an ambulance, then my husband and finally Dr. Joe. Through the panic, there is clarity, a calmness and rationalization that comes over me and drones on in my head "you are not in any pain, and there are no clots." Surely, if I was in the process of miscarrying my twins at 14 weeks, I would be experiencing both. From that moment on, I am vocalizing that fact over and over again. The ambulance comes and I now only have on my mini-dress with towels between my legs and wrapped all around me. Not my finest fashion moment! One of the girls gets into the ambulance with me and Dr. Joe calls. I tell him where I am going and that I am in no pain at all and I have no clots at all. He remains calm and I am off to the hospital. Once at the hospital, nurses and doctors asks me a barrage of questions, checking me out physically but hold off on administering a sonogram at that point, which will be the defining moment.

Marty arrives at that hospital and he is in full panic mode. Everyone is. At this point both his family and mine know what's happening but have no additional details. We are all just waiting and praying.

Emergency rooms are a strange place to be... the black hole of health care; all different types of people, with varying ailments, lying around staring at each other and waiting, and waiting, and waiting. It is the wait that is so agonizing.

Finally, three doctors come in, two of whom are interns and are being directed by the doctor who is standing right there. Let me be brutally honest here, I have a real problem with interns examining me, asking questions about what they are doing as they do it; while I am laying there worrying about my babies. Well, what happens next is gross and unfortunately you need to hear it. So, as I am being examined by an intern she is constantly looking to the doctor, who is standing right next to her, for direction. I hear him say go ahead and remove that... and then I feel a gush of warm liquid come pouring out of me. Oh my goodness - more blood. The look on her face was one of sheer panic. Before my husband had a coronary I immediately asked if they had removed a blot clot and they reply yes, I then ask if it is possible that the blood clot was formed as a result from my bleeding that day and nothing more serious, they again reply yes. Completely fed up with their abysmal bedside manner, I finally retort it would have been helpful for them to relay that information to us, instead of leaving us in the dark believing that the worst was happening. And with that, they leave and we are back to waiting.

Finally after the elapse of another 2 ½ hours, a doctor walks in and informs me that I am going to be given a sonogram. This will once and for all determine that my babies are fine. They begin the procedure and once the wand is correctly positioned I immediately see my little peanuts wiggling and moving around. My uterus is just fine, no tears, or any glaring problems. They can't explain what it is I just experienced but everything seems to be just fine. They recommend bed rest for the remainder of the week and I start to get dressed. Marty looks like the weight of the entire universe has been lifted off his shoulders. We leave the emergency room and head home. His parents drive us and we are all quietly and privately thanking God for looking after my Angels.

Marty's Thoughts:

After everything we have been through, to receive a phone call from one of Jen's coworkers informing me to what had happened, just leveled me. I was on my dinner break at work and literally raced across town to the hospital. Yes, I was in full panic mode. Remember, ER doctors are not specialists. I believed nothing of what they said and waited patiently for the OBGYN. After 2 1/2 hours of me pacing the hall way they finally showed up. Thanks are in order to my mom for sitting in the room with Jen the whole time. When I saw the babies moving around in that ultrasound I broke out in tears. The weight of the world was just lifted off our shoulders. Luckily, the worst day of my life would have a happy ending.

Steady As She Goes

For the next couple of weeks I will not leave the house without an overnight maxi pad on, just in case! I am walking, climbing and living at a snail's pace because I am petrified. Marty and I have sworn off sex until the babies are safely delivered. During my next OB appointment Dr. Joe suggests that I get a sonogram done at the hospital so he can measure my cervical length. It is at that time that I am told that my son is pushing down on my cervix and causing it to shorten; at that appointment my cervical length is 2.5. Now, I don't know much about cervical lengths but I do know that 2.5 is not very long. Dr. Joe arranges to meet with Marty and I to talk about our options and it is decided that I should go on bed rest for the remainder of my pregnancy. That was about December 4th, 2008. I am not even given the option of packing up my desk. I email everyone at my office to notify them that I am down for the count. And so it begins.

We start the process of turning the bedroom into my all-access area. I have my computer, books, magazines, phone and key beauty products all within an arm's reach. Marty and his parents begin to bring me food in bed and I start doing my Christmas shopping online. While all of this is taking place my father-in-law is quite insistent that I just be admitted to the hospital and put on hospital bed rest until the babies are born. One week goes by and I return to the hospital for another sonogram. My cervix now measures 1.2. As I prepare to return home Dr. Joe tells me that he is going to confer with a couple of colleagues about this measurement and call me. The next day Dr. Joe calls me and tells me that I am being admitting to the hospital…that day and need to get there immediately. There's a bed waiting for me. That was December 12th, 2009 at 11am. By 1pm I was at New York Presbyterian Hospital to begin my stay on hospital bed rest.

Watching the Ships Go By

I have always said that it is the little things that make me happy and I have always found happiness from the little things in the life. My side of the room is situated by the window and I am on the East River, so I have a nice view and I get to see all the big boats sailing by. And since I am claustrophobic the view doesn't make me feel so cooped in. I also have no roommate yet. My nurse, Tolighta, makes her appearance and writes her name on a white board. I have a TV that I have to pay for (daily!), a closet and a night table with a drawer and cabinet. I have a side table that swings across for when I am eating or on the computer. The nurses work in 12 hour shifts for three days in a row and then they are off. I hook up my TV immediately. The nurse comes in and talks me through everything. She tries to make me feel at home and she is very nice. Lunch comes soon after and it's bad! I didn't get to order lunch so I guess they gave me whatever they had left over. How can I survive for months on crap food? Marty is going to have to bring me food every day! The food lady then comes by and hands me a piece of paper which contains my food choices for the next day. I pick out my breakfast, lunch and dinner. Marty arrives and we are all (Marty, Annette and Augie) just sitting around waiting for Dr. Joe to come and download us on what's to come, what to expect, etc.

A couple of hours go by and Dr. Joe comes in and takes a seat. We are all sitting around him and he begins to tell us how the next 2-4 months are the most important because right now at 4 ½ months this would not be a viable pregnancy should I go into labor. It is imperative that I stay off my feet to alleviate all pressure on my cervix and to avoid going into labor at all costs. He tells me that he is going to give me a drug called Terbutaline, which is used as a fast-acting bronchodilator, often used as a short-term asthma treatment, but it can also be used as a treatment for premature labor by stopping contractions, although this use is not approved by the FDA. He goes on to tell us that twice a day nurses will check for any contractions happening and will monitor the babies heartbeats; and that every two weeks I will have a sonogram done. I am feeling deflated and I realize that I hate the term "viable" or in my case not viable. I totally understand where he is coming from but I have two babies in my belly for 4 ½ months and I have been through so much to get to this point in my life. Please do not tell me that they are not viable when in fact they are the most viable beings in the entire universe, to us. Dr. Joe, Annette and Augie leave and it's just Marty and I. Finally it's time for Marty to leave too. He starts to cry and tells me that he can't leave me, but I encourage him to go. As soon as Marty leaves it's time for Jennifer to have her meltdown. I am a maelstrom of emotions at this point, abject terror and disappointment intermingled with determined hope for positive outcome. Thank goodness I don't have a roommate! I bawl my eyes out and then eventually I fall into a fitful sleep.

A New Day, A New Routine

In my experience when you're faced with challenging situations it's always best to just create a new routine for yourself as soon as possible. A good friend once told me to "stay out of your head, it's a bad neighborhood" and they were 100% right. Develop a new routine and keep yourself busy. Time will pass and you will develop a new groove and suddenly you'll realize that you've adapted to your new life.

So that's exactly what I did the very next day. I got up about 7am and I opened my blinds and made my bed, next I washed my face, brushed my teeth, put on deodorant and freshened myself up the best I could. Then while in bed I put on my moisturizer and turned on WPIX news and that is how I started every day of the remainder of my hospital stay. That was my new routine. At about 8am every morning, give or take 15-20 minutes, breakfast would be served, and I have to tell you that the hospital food was no longer horrible. Of course my choices were limited, and the portions small, but I did order two of certain things and that helped. All in all it really wasn't so bad, but then again I am the girl who liked her cafeteria food growing up. Go figure. That is how each day started at New York Presbyterian Hospital until March 9th, 2009. More on THAT date later.

So now let's throw the nurses into mix. Every morning around 8:30am or so, an aide would come in to take my blood pressure and temperature. Then the nurse would come and generally you would have the same nurse for a couple of days. She would check for the babies heart beat and then put me on the monitor for an hour (twice a day) to check for any contractions. I had the Terbutaline placed in my leg, which is a long stick like needle that goes into your leg and is connected to a pump so whenever I had to go the bathroom or when I did shower there was a big pump attached to an IV holder cam with me. Every 24 hours a new syringe was put in and every 3 days they switched legs. Fun.

I will say that being on hospital bed rest does have its perks especially in comparison to home bed rest. Don't believe me? For starters, when you're in the hospital people definitely take notice and you get more visitors. There is a certain, "oh my goodness, she's in the *hospital*" reaction. Your food is guaranteed every day at the same time, so you don't have to rely on family and friends to bring all your meals. That is a huge inconvenience for all of them. The TV is perfectly positioned for your viewing pleasure. Your bed adjusts to all different levels for maximum comfort and your every need is met by 24 hour supervision. Not to mention the fact that you can get a haircut, manicure/pedicure, facials and visits from dogs to lift your spirits—all this from your bed side ☺ After the first week, I had my routine down and I was master of my domain!

Somebody Please Bring Me a Quarter Pounder with Cheese!

I have to be honest and say that being in the hospital for Christmas Eve, Christmas Day and New Year's Eve is definitely a buzz kill, BUT you get through it and quite frankly IF I had stayed at home on New Year's Eve it is very unlikely that I would have been up until Midnight anyway! Plus we have something great to celebrate as we enter January 1st 2009; I am approaching the 27th week of my pregnancy, and that is great news! Every additional week that I can achieve without premature labor is important. In addition to the Terbutaline they also gave me steroid shots which are administered once per day for two days for the express purpose of strengthening the babies' lungs should they be delivered early. Every precaution was being taken for me and my Angels.

Of course, my path is always rife with various obstacles and my next one arrived at week 28 weeks, in the form of my Gestational Diabetes (high blood sugar condition) test. Every woman must take this test regardless of age, ethnic background, history of diabetes, etc. This is primarily due to the fact that the pregnancy itself can precipitate the onset of Diabetes in women. For most women and most of the time the Diabetes goes away immediately after child birth and when the Placenta is passed. However, Gestational Diabetes during pregnancy if not monitored closely can be extremely dangerous. So how is the test administered? The nurse woke me up rather early, I believe it was 6am, although I'm not sure that time matters, in any case she gave me a sugar solution that contains 50 grams of glucose. The stuff tastes like a very sweet soda pop (it comes in cola, orange, or lime flavor), and you have to get all of it down in five minutes. Some hospitals/offices keep it chilled or let you pour it over ice and drink it cold.

An hour later, the nurse took a blood sample from my arm to check my blood sugar level. The idea is to see how efficiently my body processes sugar. Results should be available in a few days. If the reading is abnormal (too high), which happens 15 to 23 percent of the time, your practitioner will have you come back for a three-hour glucose tolerance test to see if you really do have gestational diabetes. The good news is that most women whose screening test shows elevated blood sugar don't turn out to have gestational diabetes.

The good news in my case is that I did not have to get the three-hour glucose tolerance test, but the bad news is I didn't need the test because my levels were so high there was no mistaking the fact that I had Gestational Diabetes. I am now informed that Gestational Diabetes is a very common side effect of taking Terbutaline.

With the verdict of definite Gestational Diabetes, the hospital sends a Diabetes specialist to meet with me as well as a Nutritionist. This place does not mess around. The Diabetes specialist informs me that I will need to have my Blood Sugar levels checked twice a day; once in the morning and once before I go to sleep. The Nutritionist tells me that I now have to start counting Carbohydrates and I will be receiving a special Diabetes menu to order my meals from. My love of food has just taken a terrible and horrific turn for me. I am so sad.

Gestational Diabetes is without question a Foodie's complete buzz kill. Given the fact that I hopefully have weeks ahead of me before I deliver my Angels, the thought of not eating whatever I want is quite frankly—very depressing, especially when viewed in the context that I also cannot move around as I would have liked as well. On the upside, not eating whatever I want could be a good thing for me. Lately, my cravings have been quite interesting to put it kindly. For example, I am not a dessert person and hadn't eaten desserts, any dessert in years, but now when it comes to dessert - specifically Sundaes, I have developed a daily obsession for them. Fast food has become a very good friend of mine as well as indulging in huge Italian submarine sandwiches and chocolate - don't even get me started on chocolate!!! I never ate chocolate and now it's like I can't live without it!

So now not only do I get pricked numerous times a day, but my meal times have been slashed to bits and pieces—leaving me with boring and bland food choices. The only silver lining I suppose I have is that maybe now I won't gain the 75+ pounds that I would have without the restrictions to my diet. Time will tell. But what was very definite was that poor Marty was no longer allowed to eat his meals in front of me at all!

Weekly Review

After being in the hospital for five weeks now, I can confidently say that I have my new routines in place and I absolutely have my hospital groove on. My daily routines don't change very much with the exception that weekends are a bit quieter and I guess seem a bit lonelier than the week nights, but I'm in good spirits and why shouldn't I be? I have my two Angels cooking inside of me and getting stronger with each passing day. I am now at 28 weeks, a feat that my Obstetrician later told me he did not think I would get to. I have a steady stream of visitors and I pretty much have my Aunt Theresa, my mother-in-law and my best friend in the world (along with her daughter) visiting me on weekends, and that definitely helps. I also must, must, must give a huge shout out to A&E and CSI: Miami along with every network that plays the Law & Order franchises in re-run. They saved me! It was actually my hospital bed rest that got me hooked on CSI: Miami. At the very least my sanity was preserved and I had a little bit of an imaginative escape from the tedium of my interminable hospital stay.

29 Weeks

I'm still early on but I'm in a really good place. I know my doctor and family are breathing a sigh of relief that I am at 29 weeks and it seems so far that my cervix is staying at .2 which is frightfully small since most women, I believe have a cervix length of maybe 5 inches. I have made friends with all the nurses and they all love Marty! The nurses here are actually exceptional human beings and I can't say enough about them, I am so grateful to have had each of them in my life during this time. It can be said that I am sort of the mayor of my hospital floor since I have been there for the longest, consistent time. It's at about 29 weeks that I also get my pedicure which boy oh boy did I need. My feet were a mess.

The remainder of my stay is basically more of the same. As each week goes by, we all feel so lucky and grateful to be where we are in this pregnancy. I can't describe in words how incredibly lucky I feel to have Dr. Joe and to be in what I feel is the most capable hands ever!!

Marty's Thoughts:

At this point, I have worked at Lincoln Center for 20 years, but never once rode a bus in the city. The Q66 bus would become my new car because it literally takes me from my job to the hospital almost door to door. Being a resident of the West Side, the East Side was all new to me. I found a cool diner on 1st Ave that would serve as Jen's escape from hospital food, even though she claimed to love it. There was also a McDonalds and Subway nearby. I also learned the ins and outs of the hospital, service elevators, shortcuts, etc. Remember, Jen spent 3 months in this place and of that entire period, I missed maybe 2 or 3 days. It became pretty routine after a while, work-hospital-work-home, and to the hospital on my days off. Since Jen was by the window, my chair overlooked the East River and Roosevelt Island. The view at times could be very breathtaking. I would often nap in that chair and even had my own hospital blanket to keep me warm. The nurses were nice, and yes, Jen did sort of become mayor of the wing. And yes, that hospital blanket is on my bed as I type this. Call me a sentimental fool.

March 9th, 2009

The day started off much like every other day. I took a shower, I ate my breakfast and I had my vitals done. At about 11:30am, the nurse came to take me for my weekly sonogram. After the sonogram I waited around for a few minutes and then the nurse told that Dr. Joe wanted to speak with me...clearly not a good sign. I took the phone and Dr. Joe very calmly told me that Sophia wasn't getting enough embryonic fluid and that it was best to take the babies out. I was 34 weeks pregnant. I called my husband and told him, He was at his parents' house doing laundry and he told his dad that he had to go because the babies were coming; I don't think it was completely registering with him. I can say that he flew to the hospital from Bayside, Queens in 25 minutes. I continued to make my other necessary calls to my mother-in-law and my aunt, my Nanny, etc.

Everyone flew to be by my side. It wasn't until much later in the day that our Angels came. By 6pm, I was wheeled to the delivery floor and prepping had started. Dr. Joe came to see me and gave me a blow by blow of what I could expect and then it explained to me about the epidural and then it started. They wheeled me into the delivery room and I sat on the table facing Dr. Joe told me to sit very still and the epidural was administered.

Then I lay down on the table with and a blue sheet separated me from the doctors. The sheet was hung from a rod and was place near my chest line. At that point they let Marty in and he stood beside. He was able to see over the sheet if we wanted to, which he did once and that was more than enough to satisfy his curiosity. It was 7:30pm and Dr. Joe asked me who I would like delivered first Michael and Sophia, I immediately answered Michael and then at 7:31pm Sophia was lifted out. Michael and Sophia were born at 7:30pm and 7:31pm on March, 9th 2009. Sophia weighed 3lbs. 9oz. and Michael was 4lbs. 12oz. Our babies were here!

Marty's Thoughts:

This was the 1st and only sonogram that I missed in three months. We had a lot of laundry to do and Jen agreed with me that I should skip this one and get that done. When she called, I could immediately tell that something was wrong. What happened next will go down in history as remarkable. Jen said Sophia was not getting enough fluid, so Dr. Joe was taking the babies out today. I took about a minute to process this before I realized that after today I would be a father. I made it from my parents' house to our house to the hospital in 25 minutes. Then, the madness ensued. Everyone was there, my parents, Jen's Aunt, etc... They all told me I could not hold the kids unless I got a manicure, so I found a place close by on 1st Ave and got one. By 7pm I was in my scrubs pacing a desolate hallway waiting for the nurse to usher me into the delivery room. All went well and our kids were brought into the world. When the nurse said I could take pictures, I left the protective curtain to do so. I must say that nothing beats seeing your wife's organs lying on a table next to her. When Dr. Joe was closing Jen up, he suggested that I should go tell the family. We all took turns going down to the NICU to see the kids. When the *smoke cleared and everyone left, I said my goodbye to Jen and went home to get much needed sleep. Outside the hospital, I looked up at the window where my kids were, got very emotional, and said to myself "you're a father now."*

Part Three

THE FANTASTIC FOUR

Introducing Michael and Sophia

After every deep valley and mountainous peak that I had lived through over the past couple of years, my babies are finally here. Immediately after delivery my little angels are taken directly to the Neo Natal Intensive Care Unit (NICU) due to the fact that they were premature and needed the special care that was imperative to help them thrive. As scary as it sounds that my babies had to be in the NICU, I am reassured that they are being well cared for and that they are not suffering from any acute medical distress. As Dr. K and the nurses explained to me this was the ideal environment with the best trained staff that limits stress to infants and meets their basic needs of warmth and nutrition to ensure their proper growth and development. Soon thereafter they wheel me into the recovery room, and although I am battling extreme nausea I am still in a state of euphoria. Marty comes into the room right away and his obvious and palpable joy is fantastic to behold. He kisses me and tells me how proud he is of me. My Aunt and Nanny arrive soon after, followed by my mother-in-law and everyone is telling me that they saw the babies who are beautiful and what a good job I had done delivering them. I have not seen my babies yet, but I still feel practically overpowered by the nausea and unable to even concentrate on that fact. Fortunately, the nurses come in soon after and give me something to stop the nausea. As I lay on the hospital bed in this empty recovery room, I have four words running in a loop around in my head I am a mom over and over again and I am so indescribably happy. I close my eyes and I just rest because I know that the ride of my life is about to begin.

A little later that evening I was wheeled back into my hospital room and Dr. Joe stops by to let me know that Michael and Sophia were both doing very well. He also provides the details about their weights and heights, I am happy to hear that they are doing well but I am so overwhelmingly tired that very soon after he departs I fall into a deep sleep.

Marty's Thoughts:

I had a chance to go to the NICU to see my children but felt extremely guilty that Jen could not. After a brief visit, I went up to the recovery room and stayed with Jen. I remember it being dark and Jen drifting in and out of awareness. Once the nausea went away they took her back to her room. I thought that it was weird that after 3 months of bein in one room, they moved her to another for the remaining 3 days of her hospital stay. I distinctly recall walking out of the hospital after midnight, standing outside and looking up at the window of the NICU and saying to myself, "My children are up there." It was such a surreal feeling.

This is UTTERly Fantastic!

The next morning the lactation specialist comes in and talks to me about breast feeding and pumping and encourages me to start pumping immediately. I had read so many books on twins and on pregnancy and I had decided from the moment that I had conceived (probably even before) that I would absolutely breastfeed. The main benefit of breast milk is by far a nutritional one. This is because the breast milk contains exactly the right balance of fatty acids, water, lactose, and amino acids that the baby needs. They say that breast milk also contains at least 100 ingredients that cannot be replicated in infant formula. Babies also cannot be allergic to their mother's milk, only have a reaction to something that the mother eats. By simply eliminating that food from her diet, the baby's reaction will clear itself up. The breast milk contains all of the nutrients that the baby needs for at least the first six months of its life and it is the most important part of their diet past this, supplying half of their nutrients up to their first birthday and a third up to their second birthday. The colostrum, or the first milk that the baby receives after being born, is a nutritional powerhouse, and is vital for helping to protect the baby against infection. The colostrum, at least for me, was more yellow in color and it isn't a whole lot. Sadly, when I was trying to get the hang of pumping, I wasted a little bit of the Colostrum and it totally bummed me out. Luckily in no time I was a breast pumping pro and I was pumping milk for the nurses to bring to Michael and Sophia. By the next day I was able to be wheeled down to finally meet my children. wow. What an unbelievably surreal feeling it was the very first moment when I saw my TWO babies in their incubators. They were right next to each other in the room. Sophia's incubator was first and she was lying on her stomach with her tiny butt in the air. It was too adorable. They took her out and gave her to me. The nurse asked if I wanted to feed her since it was time for her to eat and I eagerly said yes. Sophia latched on immediately and was sucking away!

Next it was my son's turn and it was apparent from the beginning that my son suffered from *White Boy Syndrome*, which is basically that he suffers from laziness. It was quite the task to get him to latch on and work a little. It is more work for a baby to milk from their mother's nipple than a bottle and he was having none of it. I had to consider pumping into bottles for him as much as I didn't want to. We also have to consider whether we want a super-duper high performance pumper that we can rent through the hospital and are great for heavy duty pumping, like for twins! We opted for the super-duper deluxe version and my husband even built a stand for it that could move around with me, not that I can actually move much while pumping two breasts.

Marty's Thoughts:

I was very excited to get to the hospital the next morning as I wanted to see the expression on Jen's face when she got to see our children. Michael was laying on his side, in a position just like I did. Sophia had jaundice, so she had all sorts of lamps on her, pretty much like a tanning bed. Big eye goggles covered my little peanut and I thought that this was so cute. I couldn't wait to take them all home.

Bit of a Reprieve

The day that I got released was bittersweet. I was discharged but my babies were not ready to be released yet. They wouldn't be until two weeks later. Now let me be perfectly honest here and cop to the fact that having two weeks where I could sleep in my own bed for eight hours straight, eat meals in peace and get some self-maintenance done such as dying my hair and a much needed mani/pedi was really nice and it was also a very nice reprieve before the madness that would soon define my life. Once I got home I thoroughly loved up my cat and soaked in the fact that I was part of the free world again. I'll admit being outside actually felt a little weird to me. It was time to create a new routine and so I did and it began the very next day. My days all started out with me waking up and pumping both breasts, the milk was then transferred to little pouches that were placed in a cooler bag. I then commuted into Penn Station, located on 7th and 34th street and walked to 68th and York. I would go to the Neo Natal Care Unit and visit Michael and Sophia. They were in separate incubators but right next to each other and I would transfer the milk to the refrigerator ensuring that they all were properly labeled. The reason I would bring in the milk in pouches was to ensure that the nurses had my breast milk to give to them when I was not there. However, I was not producing as much milk as I had hoped for so they were being supplemented with Similac Neosure. Much to my chagrin my breasts didn't get nearly as big as I had been hoping for. I was looking forward to Pam Anderson but got Paris Hilton instead. I'm exaggerating, of course. Anyway, after putting the milk in to the fridge I would then visit Sophia and start to feed her. I would time it so that I would arrive for her second feeding of the day. After Sophia, I would attempt to feed Michael. While I was successful on some days on other days I was not. In that case he would get the bottle with my breast milk. After feeding them and spending some time with them they would go down for a nap and I would go into the waiting room and nap too.

Generally, I was there for two feedings and then I would go home and relax. I had a C-Section when I delivered them, so I was still a bit sore and all the walking while helping me did make me a bit sorer at times. That was pretty much my routine for two weeks and then Miss Sophia was released. I can't tell you how beyond nervous we were taking her home. We brought in clothes and her car seat and an additional piece for the seat that took up more room and allowed for my tiny little angel to be as snug as she could be. I sat in the back seat with her and I think Marty probably drove 40mpg the entire way home. Looking back it was pretty hilarious and most likely standard form for all new parents. My little man, however, was not ready to be released yet, and Marty being the amazing man/dad that he is would go to the hospital and stay over with him so he would not be alone. I was home with Sophia settling into motherhood. Two days after Sophia came home, Michael was home. We were all home. Wow...

Marty's Thoughts:

I remember walking Jennifer out of the hospital after 3 months inside. I was eagerly awaiting her reaction to the outdoors. All I could think about was how good Jen was going to sleep because she would be in her own bed. It turns out that after 3 months in a reclining, soft, hospital bed, our bed was uncomfortable. I believe she slept on the couch the first couple of nights to adapt to normal life again. Sophia came home first. I remember something one of my friends told me. He said wait until you are at home and the babies start to cry. There are no more nurses to help you. He was right. Sophia would be in her bassinet crying while Jen and I looked at each other and said, "what do we do now??" I went back the next day to stay with my son. He had his circumcision, and then I sat by a window facing the 59th street bridge and held him all day. My boy and I watched the Roosevelt Island tram going back and forth. This was a great day for me. Just me and my boy. My son. The next day my father and I went in and brought Michael home. My dreams of becoming a parent and having my own family had finally come true.

WAAAAAAAAAAAA

Okay, I have both kids home now and I'm going to be brutally honest here...in my opinion and this is probably because my kids were preemie, I would say that for the first 8 months I felt more like a robotic caregiver than a mother. Marty and I handled every feeding together except when he was at work and then his mom would come over and help. Michael and Sophia were so tiny that you could not hold them the typical way and feed them, and since I could not get them to breast feed at the same time they would have my breast milk for a couple of feedings and then the Similar for the others. They would sit on our laps and we would feed them and when it came time for burping we would lean them over an open palm and gently pat their back. They weren't in my arms in a glider nestled to my breasts or with bottles. It seemed very detached and cold the way we did it, but it was necessary for their size and because there were two of them and it was imperative to me that they be on the same feeding schedule, which in the long run would definitely preserve my sanity! We fed them about every 2-3 hours, getting up in the middle of the night and walking to the kitchen to get everything ready, basically in fog. I was so exhausted that I sometimes felt wired and literally like I was running on fumes. I don't think there is any way to prepare for this level of complete exhaustion that every parent undergoes when caring for their newborn baby or babies in my case.

I did establish a routine to assist me in getting through the day whereby I showered each and every morning after their 7am feeding. I would then have some coffee and just relax. When they woke up for their next feeding I would also dress them. I had received so many outfits that I almost felt obliged to have them dressed up every day. I would actually be happy if they spit up because that would mean that I could put on a new outfit. My mother in law would come over every day at about 8am and we would sit at the table, drink coffee and talk. At that time we had acquired an additional cat and one of them shed quite a bit, so I insisted on having someone come in to clean the house every week; my justification for this expense being for the sake of the babies (wink, wink). I was also ordering groceries from Fresh Direct on a weekly basis since it was difficult for me to go food shopping with the two of them. I had a pretty steady stream of friends coming over to visit especially on the weekends so I was pretty much just settling into my routine and adjusting to motherhood.

As the days grew hotter and the kids got a bit older keeping them on a schedule was not only important to me but to them too, and God help me if I did not feed them at the exact same time. The blood curdling screams were just awful. It came to the point that I felt that my day was completely dictated by their feeding schedule, feeding them and then preparing for the next feeding, over and over again. It was my biggest challenge as it translated into me feeling pretty much cooped up in the house all day. I finally managed to figure out a method to get them both outside and into the massive double stroller I had, but it wasn't easy. First, I lugged the stroller outside (and this stroller is very heavy) and opened it up. Then I put Michael in the swing while I put the Baby Bjorn on me. Then I put Sophia in the Baby Bjorn and because the swing was higher than being on the floor, I was then able to bend over and grab Michael out of the swing. I would lock up and be on my way. Sometimes, though, it was so hot outside that I just couldn't walk around that much. When it was just unbearable outside we just stayed in and played. I was in a lot. I was feeling locked up and very lonely...

Marty's Thoughts:

In the beginning, we fed the kids every three hours so I would set my alarm clock at three hour intervals. It was tough because I did not have paternity leave and I still worked very long hours and also got up to help Jen with the feedings. I basically didn't sleep at all during this period.

This was also the only time the babies slept in their bassinets. God bless our cats. Our oldest, Jezebel, would lie at the foot of the bed and keep an eye on the children. Our kitten, Smudge, would sleep outside our bedroom door and stand guard. No one could ever tell me that animals are not smart!

S.O.S

At some point with the ingestion of all these pills, shots and other foreign substances into my body, my hormones were completely out of whack and this manifested with me becoming a psychotic raging bitch. Sounds a bit extreme, but it is the only way to explain my complete inability to moderate or filter my emotional reaction and responses. In my defense, Marty was working all day just about every day and my in laws were back and forth between the Hamptons and Queens. In any case, I was raging, and it was not good. The slightest provocation would set me off and I was extremely angry all of the time. Obviously, this was not good environment either for the babies or for my marriage. It especially made life more difficult for Marty, because on the one hand I know he felt guilty for not being there during the day and because I was also fighting with his parents, thus making for an awkward situation.

We all have expectations of others and when they don't live up to them it annoys us, but at some point you do have to ask yourself if your expectations are realistic ones that people can actually live up to. A major component of growing up and maturing is learning to accept people, including their inherent defects, and loving them in spite of it all. Another important aspect of maturity is communicating effectively with people.

That is, speaking to others in a manner in which they will be receptive to your message. This was a huge problem for me. I had a tendency to hold things in, let them fester into a nice huge ball of rage and then explode on people, like a volcano spewing vulgar language and biting remarks. It was then no surprise that these same individuals had no interest in listening to what I had to say. I was making them immediately defensive and the entire situation far worse than it ever needed to be. Any credible emotion or feeling that I may have had was immediately negated by my appalling delivery.

During this period I would have daily wars with my in-laws and this of course added even more of a burden to my husband who I was literally forcing to choose sides. As time went on the relationship degenerated to the point where we weren't even on speaking terms and the entire family was divided and strained. Looking back now, it was so incredibly sad especially given the fact that before the kids arrived we all got along so well. My MIL and I were inseparable. As time went on and the kids were almost 8 months old I recognized that this situation was completely untenable and a change was needed, one that absolutely had to start with me.

Through this experience I learned that life is not always black & white, sometimes it's downright gray and it's really hard to make sense out of things or to have a clear perspective especially when you are neck deep in it all.

Marty's Thoughts:

This was a very tough period, coupled with the fact that the kids hardly slept at night and almost never slept in their bassinets. Yes it was tough on me as a husband, a father and a son, but I knew what Jen was going through so I rode it out. Every family has its high and low points and it's just a matter of surviving the low ones.

Little White Pill to the Rescue!

Finally, after even I could no longer tolerate myself I went to my ob/gyn and he prescribed for me a pill that would help with my hormones and get me back on track.

I cannot even begin to stress how vital this information is and I want all women to really grasp the full import of what I am saying in this short section. There is no shame in taking something to take the edge off. I know that as mothers we are expected to be strong, invincible and able to bounce back quickly from any adversity or life changes. As women, new mothers, especially new mothers of multiples, our hormones will be raging, we will be sleep deprived, under fed, and feeling insecure about everything. If you need to take something to help even you out, do it. As soon as I called my doctor, he did not hesitate to prescribe something for me and I immediately felt relief. I felt calmer. My husband and I definitely had issues with his parents but I was learning to keep things in perspective and filter my feelings more. It was a great relief.

Now, the tricky thing about anti-depressants is that you really shouldn't drink wine with them. After a couple of incidents of being "over served" while taking the pills I decided that my hormones were in a good place and I stopped taking them. Wine won! At this point the kids were just about ready to celebrate their FIRST birthday and momma was getting ready to go back to work. fun times, indeed!

Have I Been Released From a Cage or What?

Finally, the time had come for me to resume work and fortunately for me, a maternity fill-in position had opened up at the cable network channel, HISTORY. So off to work I went. At this point, I had found a daycare being run out of someone's house just three blocks from our house and on the way to the LIRR. So I would drop the kids off at 7:30am and pick them up at 6pm, two days a week. I also had my best girl, Nicole, who went from being my mother's helper to my Nanny watching them for two days a week and finally Marty handling Daddy duty on Mondays - so my week was covered. However, as amazing as Nicole was she was only 19 years old and taking care of twins all day long was difficult. Eventually, my MIL began helping out and watching them 3-4 days a week. It was definitely a juggling act but we did it.

Being at home with my twins for their entire first year was thrilling, nerve racking and fulfilling, however being back at work was great! And ladies this is nothing to feel in any way guilty about. Socializing with adults was awesome, so awesome that sometimes I would tell my MIL I had to work a bit late and grab a drink with some girls from the office. Now, when I say work late I would only be home about 30 minutes later than usual. It was as if I was trying to cram all of my fun into those extra few minutes before I went home to assume all of the responsibilities of caring for my little ones. It was definitely an adjustment and quite honestly life is about adjustments and I continue to grown and learn. The one thing that I know for certain is that my babies saved me and they continue to motivate and inspire me to be the best person I can be. Thank you Michael and Sophia; mommy loves you beyond measure! ☺

EPILOGUE

I cannot tell you how important writing this book was to me. I definitely know my character defects and one of them (and there are many!) is that I'm not very disciplined and I have virtually no will power, but with this book it was different. Michael & Sophia will be six years old this March (2015), and I have finally completed this book. It was a long road but a story worth telling. As women, we endure so much, sacrifice a lot, love completely and care for our family unconditionally and it's such a shame that so many women struggle and have such difficulty trying to conceive, or are just not able to conceive at all, despite their best efforts. This story was about my journey to start a family, the one thing that meant everything to me. I did not waver and I did not give up because in every fiber of my being I knew that one day I would have my Michael and my Sophia, and they are the most important things in my life and my most significant accomplishment.

The subsequent journey that followed after they were born of course had its ups and downs. After all, I am a fulltime working mom juggling a lot, but like millions of other moms out there, I'm doing it. I have continually learned invaluable lessons from my children; the biggest one being the need to adjust certain character traits in response to those around you.

Generally changing who you are as person and ameliorating character defects that need to be fixed is often times really hard to do especially when someone is forcing you to. However, for my children I have found it easy to fix what's broken to ensure that I can be the very best mother that I can be. I'm happy to say that I have the best relationship with my in-laws, who are beyond the best Grandparents and 100% involved in their lives! I can honestly say that Motherhood continues to be a truly humbling experience.

Thank you for reading this and I sincerely hope there is something from my journey that can encourage those of you who would consider IVF to go ahead and take the plunge because it is worth it in the end. However, I want you to venture into this journey with your eyes open to the potential pitfalls and be aware of the different protocols available to you, so that you can have the family you always dreamed of.

Jenn's Glossary

IVF – In Vitro Fertilization - a viable alternative to for those of us who cannot have a baby without assistance. With this an egg and sperm are fertilized manually in a laboratory dish, and once the fertilization is successful the embryo is physically inserted into the uterus. This is just a basic sketch of the process, there is of course a bevy of other factors that one must take into account to go from this to actually becoming impregnated successfully.

Beta blood test – there are two types, qualitative and quantitative. The qualitative tests are usually not used since results from it are practically the same as those from the more sensitive home pregnancy tests that use urine.

For the quantitative test, the amount of hCG in your blood is measured and expressed as a numerical level. These tests are usually used for women like me who are having fertility treatments or are under a doctor's care as she is trying to get pregnant. Essentially, we have several of these tests to make sure that our hCG levels are increasing over time.

Human Chorionic Gonadotropin (**hCG**) is a hormone produced during pregnancy that is made by the developing placenta after conception.

Micro Flare- So since I was on the Lupron protocol, taking those birth control pills on time every day as directed, the micro-flare protocol seems to part of this procedure. In an effort to stimulate the ovaries to make eggs, it somehow works with the body when Lupron first releases the body's own FSH hormone prior to suppressing the ovaries. There is a lot more to this entire process that you will need to discuss in detail with your doctor, unlike me to know exactly what you are getting in to.

Stimming – after the flare comes the long process of stimming which can last anywhere from eight to fourteen days. You get stuck with a needle every day to put various hormones into your body to stimulate your ovaries to produce multiple eggs. At each visit, your doctor's office will draw blood to study the changes in your hormones and in some cases a vaginal ultrasound will be performed to check on the progress of your follicles. Just be prepared to be BLOATED all the time as you are required to drink lots and lots of liquids – no caffeine though, and you will feel tired all of the time, no matter how much you sleep as well.

FSH number (Follicle Secreting Hormone) - FSH is responsible for promoting and sustaining ovarian follicular growth in females. FSH regulates the development, growth, pubertal maturation, and reproductive processes of the body. If you are undergoing the IVF process, you want this number to be under twelve, the lower the number the better the quality of your follicles.

Antagonistic Protocol – The antagonist medications that are used stops the eggs from being released before you manually trigger their release, although Lupron also prevents the eggs premature release, this protocol is more aggressive.

About the Author

Jennifer Prudenti is a mother of two beautiful kids, Sophia and Michael, and she lives in Albertson, NY with her husband, Marty, their children and the family cats, Smudgie and Sabrina. She is a mother, daughter, wife, friend, co-worker -- she is just like you and her story could be anyone's. She is a marketing professional that has worked in the music business, publishing and television, and writing is her passion.

Forward by Aimee E. Raupp MS, Lac, Author or *Chill Out and Get Healthy* and *You Can Get Pregnant*

Printed in the United States
By Bookmasters